SALICYLATE SENSITIVITY
COOKBOOK

Safe and Satisfying Recipes for a Better You.

Rhonda C Anderson Ms Rdn

Table of Contents

Chapter 1: Understanding Salicylate Sensitivity

1.1 What Are Salicylates?.

Chapter 2: Navigating a Salicylate-Free Diet

Chapter 3: Essential Ingredients for a Salicylate-Sensitive Kitchen.

BONUS PAGE.

Disclaimer

Always consult with your healthcare provider before making any significant changes to your diet, especially if you have any existing health conditions. Your well-being is our top priority, and we hope this book serves as a beacon of hope and a tool for joy in

your culinary journey.

Dedication

To all the brave souls navigating the challenges of salicylate sensitivity

This book is dedicated to you. Your strength and resilience inspire us every day. You face each meal with courage, turning what could be a struggle into a journey of discovery and self-care.

You are not alone in this. Together, we stand stronger, embracing the journey towards better health and well-being.

Remember, every step you take is a testament to your incredible strength.

With all my heart,
Rhonda C. Anderson

Introduction

*Welcome to **the "Salicylate Sensitivity Cookbook"** by Rhonda C. Anderson. We're delighted you've chosen to take this important step towards a healthier and happier life. Whether you're just beginning to understand salicylate sensitivity or looking for delicious and safe meal options, this cookbook is designed with you in mind.*

Salicylate sensitivity is a condition that affects many people, often causing a range of symptoms from headaches to skin reactions. For those in the United States and around the world, finding foods that fit into a salicylate-sensitive diet can be challenging.

Historically, salicylates have been used in foods and medicines for their natural preservative qualities. While these compounds can be beneficial for many, they can cause significant issues for those who are sensitive to them.

In this cookbook, you'll find a wealth of recipes tailored to those who need to manage their salicylate intake. Rhonda C. Anderson, a seasoned professional chef and a trusted name in the culinary world, has compiled over 100 cookbooks, helping countless individuals navigate their dietary needs with joy and confidence.

Her cookbooks have sold over 80,000 copies across the USA and internationally, bringing comfort and satisfaction to many kitchens.

The ***"Salicylate Sensitivity Cookbook"*** is not just a collection of recipes; it's a comprehensive guide to living well while managing salicylate sensitivity. Inside, you'll discover a 30-day meal plan to kickstart your journey towards better health. This plan is meticulously designed to ensure you enjoy a variety of flavours and textures while keeping your diet safe and balanced. Additionally, this book offers two outstanding benefits: a guide to understanding salicylates and their effects on the body, and practical tips for sourcing and preparing low-salicylate foods that fit seamlessly into your daily routine.

We've crafted this book to make your cooking experience enjoyable and stress-free. Each recipe is thoughtfully created to be easy to follow, even for those new to cooking. Whether you're making breakfast, lunch, dinner, or a snack, you'll find options that satisfy your taste buds and support your health goals. The meals are designed to be nourishing, vibrant, and full of flavour, ensuring that you never feel deprived or limited.

Thank you for choosing this book and investing your time and money into a resource that promises to make a positive impact on your life. We understand the importance of your decision, and we assure you that you've made a wise choice. The care and expertise poured into these pages reflect years of culinary experience and a deep understanding of dietary needs. Rhonda C. Anderson's reputation for delivering practical and delightful recipes means you're in safe hands. You're joining a community of readers who have found joy and relief in her cookbooks, and your experience will be no different.

As you start exploring the recipes and meal plans, we encourage you to follow them closely. Implementing the guidance in this book will help you discover a new world of flavours that align with your dietary needs. You'll soon realise the benefits of a diet that suits your body and supports your well-being.

The cookbook is here to support you every step of the way. Enjoy the process of cooking and eating delicious, safe meals. We're confident that this book will be a valuable addition to your kitchen, bringing you health and happiness. Welcome to a new chapter of mindful and joyful eating.

Real-Life Success Stories and Tips from Salicylate Sensitivity Survivors: The Journey of Peter W. Clifford

Peter W. Clifford's life changed in ways he never imagined when he first discovered his sensitivity to salicylates. Living in a bustling city, he had always enjoyed a variety of foods and activities, never suspecting that the headaches, fatigue, and gastrointestinal issues he frequently experienced were linked to something as innocuous as the compounds found in many fruits, vegetables, and even personal care products.

For years, Peter struggled to find relief. Doctors offered various diagnoses, none of which seemed to address the root of his problems. The constant cycle of trial and error with medications and diets left him feeling more frustrated and helpless.

It wasn't until a particularly severe reaction after a family meal that a friend suggested he might be dealing with salicylate sensitivity.

This revelation was both a relief and a new source of anxiety. How could he navigate a world so rich in these ubiquitous compounds?

Enter the "Salicylate Sensitivity Cookbook" by Rhonda C. Anderson. Peter stumbled upon this book during a late-night search for answers. The title alone gave him a glimmer of hope. As he delved into the pages, he found not just recipes, but a lifeline. The book wasn't just a collection of meals—it was a guide to reclaiming his life from the grips of his sensitivity.

Rhonda's book began with detailed explanations of salicylates and their effects on the body, offering clarity on a topic that had been a source of confusion and despair for Peter. He appreciated the thoroughness with which she covered the science behind salicylate sensitivity, making it accessible and relatable. This foundation of knowledge was crucial for Peter, helping him understand his condition in a way that no medical appointment had.

But the real magic happened in the kitchen. Rhonda's cookbook was filled with recipes that transformed Peter's approach to food.

He learned how to prepare delicious, nourishing meals without fear of triggering his sensitivity. Each recipe was crafted with care, considering not just the avoidance of salicylates but also the joy of eating.

Peter was no longer resigned to bland, restrictive diets. Instead, he found himself exploring new flavours and ingredients, guided by Rhonda's inventive and thoughtful recipes.

One of his favourite dishes became the herb-roasted chicken with a side of quinoa and steamed vegetables, seasoned with Rhonda's special blend of low-salicylate herbs.

It was a revelation to Peter that he could enjoy such a flavorful and satisfying meal without any adverse effects. This dish, like many others in the cookbook, restored his confidence and excitement about food.

Beyond the recipes, the real-life success stories featured in the book resonated deeply with Peter. He read about others who had walked a similar path, their experiences mirroring his own struggles and triumphs.

These stories offered him a sense of community and understanding, which was something he had sorely missed. Knowing he was not alone in his journey was a profound comfort.

Peter also found the tips and practical advice sprinkled throughout the book invaluable. From grocery shopping strategies to dining out tips, Rhonda's guidance equipped him with the tools to navigate his everyday life with confidence.

He learned how to communicate his needs effectively in social situations and even discovered ways to manage his sensitivity in non-food contexts, like choosing salicylate-free personal care products.

In time, Peter's health improved significantly. He no longer lived in constant fear of his next meal. The debilitating symptoms that had once controlled his life became a thing of the past. The "Salicylate Sensitivity Cookbook" had not only provided him with delicious recipes but had also empowered him with knowledge and community.

Today, Peter shares his story with others, hoping to inspire and guide those who are just beginning their journey with salicylate sensitivity. He credits Rhonda C. Anderson's book with giving him the tools and confidence to take back control of his life. "This cookbook," he often says with a smile, "is more than just a collection of recipes; it's a beacon of hope."

Chapter 1: Understanding Salicylate Sensitivity

1.1 What Are Salicylates?

Salicylates are natural chemicals found in many plants, including fruits, vegetables, and herbs. They serve as a defence mechanism, protecting plants from insects and diseases. These compounds are also found in many common products, such as medications like aspirin, and in preservatives and flavourings.

When we eat foods containing salicylates or use products with these chemicals, most people can process them without any issues. However, some people are sensitive to salicylates, which can lead to a range of uncomfortable symptoms.

The Natural Chemicals in Foods and Products

Why Salicylates Matter for Your Health

Understanding salicylates is crucial for those with sensitivity. This sensitivity can cause various reactions, affecting daily life and well-being. By knowing where salicylates are found and how they affect your body, you can make informed choices to avoid discomfort and maintain better health.

For those with salicylate sensitivity, managing intake can be a game-changer. It helps in reducing symptoms and improving the quality of life. Simple changes in diet and product choices can make a significant difference. By being mindful of these natural chemicals, you can enjoy your meals and everyday activities without worrying about adverse reactions.

<u>**1.2.Signs and Symptoms**</u>

<u>**Common Reactions and Misdiagnoses**</u>

Salicylate sensitivity can present in various ways, often mimicking other conditions, which can lead to misdiagnosis. Common symptoms include headaches, rashes, stomach pain, and nasal congestion. These reactions are similar to those seen in allergies, making it tricky to identify the true cause.

Many people with salicylate sensitivity are initially diagnosed with conditions like food allergies, asthma, or even irritable bowel syndrome (IBS). Because the symptoms overlap, it's easy to mistake one condition for another. Recognizing the unique signs of salicylate sensitivity is key to finding relief and avoiding unnecessary treatments.

How to Recognize Salicylate Sensitivity

To pinpoint salicylate sensitivity, pay attention to your body's reactions after consuming certain foods or using specific products. If you notice patterns, like recurring symptoms after eating certain fruits or using particular toiletries, salicylates might be the culprit.

Keep a symptom diary to track your experiences. Note what you ate, the products you used, and any symptoms that followed. This record can be invaluable when discussing your health with a professional and can help identify salicylate sensitivity as a potential issue.

1.3.Causes and Risk Factors

Genetic Predispositions and Lifestyle Triggers

Salicylate sensitivity often has a genetic component, meaning it can run in families. If a close relative has this sensitivity or related conditions like asthma or eczema, you might be at higher risk. However, genetics isn't the only factor at play.

Lifestyle and environmental factors also contribute to salicylate sensitivity. High exposure to salicylates through diet or personal care products can trigger sensitivity in some people. Stress, diet, and overall health status can influence how your body handles these chemicals. Being aware of your family history and lifestyle choices can help manage and mitigate risks.

How Environmental Factors Influence Sensitivity

Environmental factors, such as pollution and exposure to chemicals, can increase the risk of developing salicylate sensitivity. These elements can overwhelm the body's ability to process salicylates, leading to a buildup that triggers symptoms.

Eating a diet high in processed foods, which often contain salicylates as preservatives or flavourings, can also contribute to sensitivity. Additionally, chronic stress and poor health can lower your body's tolerance to salicylates, making you more susceptible to their effects.

1.4. Diagnosis and Testing

Effective Methods for Identifying Sensitivity

Diagnosing salicylate sensitivity involves a combination of observation, dietary changes, and testing. One effective approach is the elimination diet, where foods high in salicylates are removed from your diet for a period, and then gradually reintroduced. This helps identify which foods trigger symptoms.

Blood tests and other medical assessments can also support the diagnosis. These tests measure the body's response to salicylates and can confirm sensitivity. However, they are not always conclusive and are best used alongside dietary observations.

Working with Healthcare Professionals

Navigating salicylate sensitivity is easier with professional guidance. Healthcare providers, such as allergists or dietitians, can offer valuable insights and support. They can help design a safe and effective elimination diet, suggest alternatives to high-salicylate foods, and provide strategies for managing symptoms.

Regular consultations ensure you're on the right track and adapting well to any dietary changes. With the right support, you can effectively manage salicylate sensitivity and improve your overall quality of life.

Chapter2: Navigating a Salicylate-Free Diet

2.1. The Basics of a Low-Salicylate Diet

A.Essential Foods to Include and Avoid

Adopting a low-salicylate diet involves making some key changes to your food choices. Salicylates are naturally found in many plants and are common in foods like fruits, vegetables, and spices. For those sensitive to salicylates, eating these foods can lead to uncomfortable symptoms.

Foods to Include:

Proteins: Lean meats like chicken, turkey, and certain cuts of beef and pork are generally low in salicylates. Eggs and most fish are also safe options.

Grains: Rice, oats, and barley are excellent choices. They provide essential carbs and can be the base for many meals.

Dairy: Milk, cheese, and yoghurt can be part of your diet unless you have other sensitivities. They provide vital calcium and protein.

Vegetables: While many vegetables contain salicylates, some like potatoes, cabbage, and iceberg lettuce are low in them.

Fruits: Pears and bananas are typically well-tolerated and can be eaten fresh or as snacks.

Oils and Fats: Use canola or sunflower oil for cooking, as they are low in salicylates.

Foods to Avoid:

Fruits and Vegetables: Avoid high-salicylate foods like tomatoes, berries, and certain leafy greens such as spinach and kale.

Spices and Flavorings: Many herbs and spices, including turmeric, cumin, and cinnamon, are high in salicylates. Stick to simple seasonings like salt and sugar.

Processed Foods: Packaged snacks, ready meals, and anything with artificial flavours or preservatives can be problematic.

Beverages: Avoid drinks like fruit juices, wines, and teas, which can be high in salicylates.

Understanding which foods are safe and which to avoid is the first step to managing your diet successfully.

B.Building a Balanced, Nutrient-Rich Diet

Maintaining a low-salicylate diet doesn't mean you have to sacrifice nutrition. It's all about balance and finding alternatives that keep you healthy.

2.2.Planning and Preparing Meals

Proteins: Include a variety of meats and fish in your diet to ensure you get enough protein. Eggs are versatile and can be used in many different dishes.

Carbohydrates: Grains and cereals should be your primary source of carbohydrates. Rice and oats can be used in a multitude of ways, from breakfast porridges to hearty dinners.

Fats: Healthy fats are crucial. Canola and sunflower oils are good for cooking, and small amounts of butter or ghee can add flavour without adding salicylates.

Vitamins and Minerals: Even though you need to avoid many fruits and vegetables, you can still get essential nutrients. Potatoes and cabbage are great sources of vitamin C, while dairy products can help with your calcium intake.

Hydration: Drink plenty of water throughout the day. If you miss flavoured drinks, consider making your own flavoured water with a slice of pear or banana.

Creating a balanced, nutrient-rich diet is key to staying healthy and feeling your best on a low-salicylate plan.

A.Strategies for Successful Meal Planning

Meal planning on a low-salicylate diet might seem daunting at first, but with some organisation, it can be straightforward and stress-free.

B.Tips for Safe and Easy Meal Preparation

Weekly Planning: Start by planning your meals for the week. This not only saves time but also helps avoid the temptation to grab something quick and potentially high in salicylates.

Batch Cooking: Prepare large portions of salicylate-safe dishes that you can freeze and reheat later. This is especially helpful for busy days when you don't have time to cook.

Safe Recipes: Keep a collection of go-to recipes that you know are safe and enjoyable. This makes it easier to whip up meals without second-guessing ingredient lists.

Shopping Lists: Write detailed shopping lists based on your meal plans. Stick to your list to avoid buying foods that aren't safe for your diet.

Planning ahead ensures you always have safe, delicious options ready to go, making mealtime enjoyable and stress-free.

2.3. Eating Out and Social Situations

Preparing meals on a low-salicylate diet doesn't have to be complicated. Here are some tips to keep it simple and safe.

Separate Work Areas: If you share your kitchen with others who eat a regular diet, designate separate areas for your food preparation to avoid cross-contamination.

Simple Cooking Methods: Stick to basic cooking methods like baking, boiling, and grilling. These techniques are less likely to alter the salicylate content of your food.

Flavour Enhancements: Use safe flavourings like salt, sugar, and safe oils. Avoid spices and herbs that can be high in salicylates.

Read Labels: Always check labels when using packaged foods. Look for any hidden salicylates in ingredients lists.

Safe Utensils: Use separate cutting boards, knives, and utensils for your food to prevent accidental mixing with high-salicylate ingredients.

Dining out or attending social events can be challenging on a low-salicylate diet, but with a few strategies, you can still enjoy these experiences.

A.Navigating Restaurants and Social Gatherings

Research Ahead: Before going to a restaurant, look at the menu online. Identify safe options or call ahead to discuss your dietary needs with the staff.

Simple Dishes: Opt for simple, grilled or roasted meats and plain sides like rice or potatoes. These are more likely to be free from hidden salicylates.

Customise Your Order: Don't hesitate to ask for modifications. Most restaurants are willing to accommodate dietary restrictions if you explain clearly what you need.

Bring Your Own Snacks: For social gatherings, consider bringing a small dish or snacks that you can eat if the available food isn't suitable.

Be Prepared: Carry a list of safe and unsafe foods with you. This can be a handy reference when making decisions on the go.

B.Communicating Your Needs Effectively

Effective communication is key to managing a low-salicylate diet, especially when you're not in control of the food preparation.

Clear Explanation: When discussing your diet with others, be clear and specific. Explain which foods you can and cannot eat and why.

Positive Attitude: Approach conversations with a positive attitude. People are more likely to accommodate your needs if you're friendly and understanding.

Educate Gently: Sometimes, you might need to educate friends or family about your dietary restrictions. Do this gently, focusing on how they can help keep you safe and comfortable.

Express Gratitude: Always thank people for their efforts to accommodate your diet. This encourages them to continue being supportive.

<u>Prepare for Questions:</u> Be ready to answer questions about your diet. This can be an opportunity to help others understand your needs better.

Good communication ensures that those around you understand and support your dietary requirements, making it easier to stick to your low-salicylate diet in any situation.

Chapter3:
Essential Ingredients for a
Salicylate-Sensitive
Kitchen

3.1.Stocking Your Pantry

A.Must-Have Ingredients for Low-Salicylate Cooking

In any kitchen, the foundation of a great meal starts with what's in the pantry. When cooking with low-salicylate ingredients, the key is to have a well-stocked pantry that supports flavorful and safe dishes. Here are some must-have staples:

1.Grains and Flours: Choose low-salicylate options like white rice, oats, and millet. These grains are versatile and can be the base for many meals. For baking, stock up on white rice flour, oat flour, and potato starch.

2.Proteins: Keep a variety of low-salicylate proteins on hand. This includes fresh chicken, turkey, lamb, and fish like cod or haddock. Eggs are also a great protein source and can be used in many recipes.

3.Fruits and Vegetables: While many fruits and vegetables are high in salicylates, some safe choices include bananas, peeled pears, and green beans. Stock up on these and other low-salicylate options to ensure you have healthy sides and snacks.

4.Dairy and Alternatives: Dairy can be a tricky area. Stick with products like cream cheese, cottage cheese, and plain yoghurt, which are typically low in salicylates. If you're avoiding dairy, rice milk or coconut milk are good alternatives.

5.Fats and Oils: Choose oils like sunflower oil and canola oil for cooking. These are generally low in salicylates and can be used in a variety of ways, from frying to baking.

B.How to Replace High-Salicylate Foods

1.Spices and Seasonings: Replace high-salicylate herbs and spices like oregano and basil with safe options such as chives, parsley, and garlic powder. These alternatives will keep your dishes flavorful without adding unnecessary salicylates.

2.Sweeteners: Many sweeteners, such as honey and maple syrup, are high in salicylates. Instead, use white sugar or golden syrup. These can be used in baking and cooking without altering the taste significantly.

3.Fruits: If you're used to eating fruits like berries and apples, which are high in salicylates, try switching to bananas and peeled pears. They provide a similar texture and sweetness but are safer for a low-salicylate diet.

4.Vegetables: Substitute high-salicylate vegetables like tomatoes and cucumbers with options like potatoes, iceberg lettuce, and green beans. These can be used in salads, soups, and as side dishes.

3.2.Herbs, Spices, and Flavor Enhancers

1.Herbs: Fresh herbs like parsley, chives, and cilantro are great for adding fresh, green flavours to your dishes. They can be used in salads, as garnishes, or blended into sauces.

2.Spices: While many spices are high in salicylates, some like garlic powder and salt are safe and versatile. They can add depth and savoriness to your dishes.

3.Flavours: For a tangy twist, use lemon juice instead of lime or vinegar. Lemon juice is lower in salicylates and can brighten up salads, marinades, and desserts.

<u>4.Umami Boosters:</u> Use low-salicylate umami-rich ingredients like plain, unsweetened yoghurt or cream to add a creamy, savoury element to your cooking.

Safe Seasonings and Flavor Alternatives

B.Creating Delicious, Salicylate-Free Dishes

1.Layer Flavours: Use multiple low-salicylate ingredients to build flavour. For example, combine garlic powder, chives, and a bit of lemon juice to create a complex taste profile.

2.Texture Play: Texture can enhance the eating experience. Add crunchy elements like roasted sunflower seeds or creamy components like plain yoghourt to your dishes.

3.Experiment: Don't be afraid to try new combinations. Mix and match your safe ingredients to discover new flavours that you love.

3.3.Healthy Substitutions

A.Alternatives for Common High-Salicylate Ingredients

1.Bread: Instead of whole grain or multigrain bread, opt for white bread or bread made from safe flours like rice or potato flour.

2.Nuts: Many nuts are high in salicylates. Substitute with seeds like sunflower or pumpkin seeds, which provide a similar crunch and nutritional benefits.

3.Oils: Use sunflower oil or canola oil instead of olive oil or nut oils, which can be high in salicylates.

4.Canned Goods: Choose fresh or frozen vegetables instead of canned, as the canning process can concentrate salicylates.

B.Making Your Favourite Recipes Work for You

1.Adjust Spices: Replace high-salicylate spices with safe alternatives that offer a similar flavour profile. For example, use chives instead of oregano.

2.Swap Ingredients: Replace high-salicylate ingredients with low-salicylate options. Use white rice instead of brown rice, or peeled pears instead of apples.

3.Focus on Technique: Cooking techniques like roasting, grilling, or slow-cooking can enhance the natural flavours of low-salicylate ingredients. Experiment with different methods to bring out the best in your dishes.

3.4.Cooking Tools and Gadgets

1.Good Knives: A sharp chef's knife and a paring knife are crucial for efficient prep work. They help you chop vegetables, slice meats, and create beautiful garnishes.

2.Quality Pots and Pans: Invest in a few high-quality pots and pans. A non-stick skillet, a heavy-duty saucepan, and a sturdy roasting pan can cover most of your cooking needs.

3.Mixing Bowls: A set of mixing bowls in various sizes will make it easier to prep and mix ingredients.

4.Measuring Tools: Accurate measurements are important, especially in baking. Have a set of measuring cups and spoons, along with a kitchen scale.

5.Blender or Food Processor: These are great for making purees, sauces, and soups. They also come in handy for mixing batters or making dough.

Essential Kitchen Tools for Every Home Cook

How to Make Cooking Enjoyable and Efficient

1.Organise Your Space: Keep your kitchen organised so that everything you need is within easy reach. Group similar items together and store them in easily accessible places.

2.Prep Ahead: Spend some time each week preparing ingredients. Chop vegetables, measure out spices, and pre-cook grains so that they're ready to use when you need them.

3.Use Time-Saving Tools: Take advantage of tools like slow cookers, pressure cookers, and food processors. They can cut down on prep and cooking time.

4.Clean as You Go: Keep your workspace tidy by cleaning up as you cook. This makes the final cleanup much easier and keeps your kitchen more pleasant to work in.

Chapter4: Delicious Breakfasts and Brunches

1.Banana-Oat Cottage Cheese Pancakes

Prep Time:10 mins
Cook Time:10 mins
Total Time:20 mins
Serving=5

Ingredients

Dry Ingredients:
- ½ cup gluten-free oats
- 1 scoop protein powder (Optional)
- 2 tablespoons brown sugar
- 1 teaspoon ground cinnamon
- 1 teaspoon baking powder

<u>**Wet Ingredients:**</u>

- 1 banana
- 2 eggs
- ½ cup cottage cheese
- 1 teaspoon vanilla extract
- water as needed

<u>Directions</u>

1. Heat a griddle or a large skillet over medium heat.

2. In a blender, process the oatmeal, protein powder, brown sugar, cinnamon, and baking powder until finely ground. Transfer this mixture to a large bowl.

3. Blend the banana, eggs, cottage cheese, and vanilla extract in the blender until smooth. Combine this mixture with the dry ingredients in the bowl and stir to create a thick batter. Add water to the batter to reach your desired consistency.

4. Pour 1/4 to 1/2 cup of batter for each pancake onto the preheated cooking surface. Cook until the bottom is golden brown, about 3 to 5 minutes. Flip the pancakes and cook the other side until golden

and the centre is cooked through, another 3 to 5 minutes.

Nutritional value
Carbs=21g
Calories=150
Protein=10g
Fats=4g

2.Coconut and Cinnamon Rice Cereal.

Prep Time:5 mins
Cook Time:20 mins
Total Time:25 mins
Servings:4

Ingredients

- 1 tablespoon sweet cream butter
- ½ cup brown rice
- ½ cup coconut milk
- ½ cup water
- 2 tablespoons white sugar
- ½ teaspoon ground cinnamon

Directions

1. Heat butter in a small saucepan over medium heat until it starts to brown, approximately 2 to 3 minutes.

2. Blend uncooked rice until the grains are coarsely broken. Add the rice to the butter and cook, stirring, until it turns lightly brown, about 5 minutes.

3. In a bowl, mix coconut milk, water, sugar, and cinnamon until the sugar dissolves. Gradually pour this mixture into the rice while stirring constantly.

4. Lower the heat, cover the saucepan, and let it simmer until the rice becomes tender, roughly 20 minutes.

Nutritional value
Carbs=52g
Calories=394
Protein=7g
Fats=21g

3.Quinoa Porridge

Prep Time:5 mins
Cook Time:30 mins
Total Time:35 mins
Servings:3

<u>Ingredients</u>

- ½ cup quinoa
- ¼ teaspoon ground cinnamon
- 1 ½ cups almond milk
- ½ cup water
- 2 tablespoons brown sugar
- 1 teaspoon vanilla extract (Optional)
- 1 pinch salt

<u>Directions</u>

1. Place a saucepan over medium heat and add the quinoa. Sprinkle it with cinnamon and toast it for about 3 minutes, stirring frequently. Pour in the almond milk, water, and vanilla, then mix in the

brown sugar and salt. Bring the mixture to a boil, then reduce to low heat and simmer until the porridge thickens and the quinoa is tender, approximately 25 minutes. If the liquid evaporates before the quinoa is done, add a bit more water. Stir occasionally, particularly towards the end, to prevent sticking or burning.

<u>Nutritional value</u>
Carbs=31g
Calories=174
Protein=4g
Fats=3g

4.Spinach Omelette with Leftover Mashed Potatoes

Prep Time:5 mins
Cook Time:10 mins
Total Time:15 mins
Servings:1

<u>**Ingredients**</u>

- 1 teaspoon coconut oil
- 1 medium Spanish sweet onion, chopped
- 2 cups fresh spinach
- 2 large eggs, beaten
- 1 ounce shredded mozzarella cheese
- 1 cup leftover mashed potatoes
- 1 tablespoon salsa
- salt and ground black pepper to taste

<u>**Directions**</u>

1. In a pan, heat oil over medium-high heat. Sauté the onions until they soften, which should take about 5 minutes. Stir in the spinach and beaten eggs, ensuring they are well-coated. Sprinkle cheese on top and cover the pan with a lid.

2. Reduce the heat and let it steam until the eggs are firm, approximately 5 minutes.

3. While the eggs are cooking, heat the leftover mashed potatoes in the microwave for 1 to 2 minutes.

4. Once the omelette is ready, place it over the warmed potatoes and finish with a topping of salsa. Season with salt and pepper to your liking.

Nutritional value
Carbs=52g
Calories=520
Protein=27g
Fats=21g

5.Cinnamon-Peach Cottage Cheese Pancakes

Prep Time:10 mins
Cook Time:30 mins
Total Time:40 mins
Servings:4

Ingredients
- 4 eggs
- 1 cup cottage cheese

- ½ cup milk
- 1 teaspoon vanilla extract
- 2 tablespoons butter, melted
- 1 peach, shredded
- 1 cup all-purpose flour
- 2 tablespoons white sugar
- 1 pinch salt
- ¾ teaspoon baking soda
- 1 teaspoon ground cinnamon

<u>Directions</u>

1. In a large bowl, blend together eggs, cottage cheese, milk, vanilla, butter, and peaches. In a separate smaller bowl, mix the flour, sugar, salt, baking soda, and cinnamon. Gradually fold the dry ingredients into the cottage cheese mixture until just combined.

2. Preheat a lightly greased griddle over medium-high heat. Spoon the batter onto the griddle, allowing large spoonfuls to cook until bubbles appear and the edges become dry. Flip and cook the other side until golden brown. Repeat this process with the remaining batter.

<u>**Nutritional value**</u>
Carbs=36g
Calories=348
Protein=22g
Fats=12g

6.Quinoa Buckwheat Pancakes.

Prep Time:15 mins
Cook Time:5 mins
Total Time:20 mins
Servings:4

<u>**Ingredients**</u>
- 1 cup buttermilk
- 1 egg, lightly beaten
- 2 tablespoons canola oil
- 1 tablespoon honey
- ½ cup buckwheat flour
- ½ cup quinoa flour
- 1 teaspoon baking powder
- ½ teaspoon baking soda

- ½ teaspoon salt

Directions

1. In a large mixing bowl, combine buttermilk, egg, canola oil, and honey. In a separate bowl, blend together buckwheat flour, quinoa flour, baking powder, baking soda, and salt. Gradually incorporate the dry ingredients into the buttermilk mixture, stirring until well combined.

2. Preheat a lightly oiled griddle over medium heat. Pour 1/4 cup of batter per pancake onto the griddle. Cook for 3 to 4 minutes until bubbles appear on the surface and the edges look dry. Flip the pancakes and cook for an additional 2 to 3 minutes until the other side is golden brown. Repeat with the remaining batter.

Nutritional value
Carbs=14g
Calories=105
Protein=3g
Fats=5g

7.Homemade Plain Yogurt

Prep Time:20 mins
Cook Time:6 hrs
Total Time:6 hrs 20 mins
Servings:5

Ingredients

- 1 quart 1% milk
- ¼ cup dry milk powder
- 3 tablespoons plain yoghourts with active cultures

Directions

1.Prepare the Jars: Place a large pot on the stove and set 5 sterile half-pint canning jars inside. Fill the pot with enough water to submerge the jars up to their necks. Turn the heat to low, aiming to maintain a steady temperature between 110°F and 115°F

(45°C) for 4 to 6 hours. Use a candy or meat thermometer to check the temperature periodically.

2.Heat the Milk:In a large saucepan, combine the milk and dry milk powder, stirring until the powder is fully dissolved. Heat the mixture over medium heat until it reaches a steaming point, about 180°F (82°C) on your thermometer. Remove the pan from the heat and place it in a bowl of ice water to cool it down to 115°F (45°C).

3.Mix with Yogurt: Once the milk has cooled to the desired temperature, take about 1 cup of the milk and blend it thoroughly with the plain yoghurt. Then, stir this mixture back into the saucepan with the rest of the milk.

4.Fill the Jars: Pour the milk mixture into the warmed glass jars, leaving about 1/2 inch of space at the top. Place the jars in the warm water bath in the pot. Ensure the water level matches the level of the yoghurt inside the jars. Maintain the temperature between 110°F and 115°F (45°C) for 4 to 6 hours, preferably 6. Avoid stirring or disturbing the yoghurt during this time to prevent it from becoming watery.

5.Check the Yogurt: After the allotted time, gently press on the top of the yoghurt or tilt the jars slightly to see if the yoghurt has set. It's ready when it's firm and has a thin layer of yellowish liquid on top. Remove the jars from the water bath, dry them off, and seal them with clean lids and rings. Store the yoghurt in the refrigerator for 1 to 2 weeks.

6.Save Some Starter: Remember to keep a small amount of your homemade yoghurt as a starter for the next batch. Over time, the effectiveness of the homemade starter may diminish, so every fourth or fifth batch, consider using store-bought yoghurt labelled with "live active cultures" as a fresh starter. Enjoy your homemade yoghurt!

Nutritional value

Carbs=15g
Calories=122
Protein=11g
Fats=3g

8.Grain-Free Butter Bread

Prep Time:20 mins
Cook Time:30 mins
Additional Time:10 mins
Total Time:1 hr
Servings:8

Ingredients

- 6 large eggs
- 1 ½ cups finely ground almond flour
- 2 teaspoons baking powder
- 1 teaspoon fine salt
- ¼ cup melted butter
- ⅛ teaspoon cream of tartar

Directions

1.Separate the eggs: Gently crack each egg into your hand, allowing the whites to drip into a bowl while keeping the yolks in a separate bowl.

2.*Preheat the oven* to 375°F (190°C). Grease a loaf pan with butter and place parchment paper at the bottom.

3.Prepare the dry ingredients: In a food processor, combine almond flour, baking powder, and salt. Add the egg yolks and melted butter. Pulse until the mixture is well blended, scraping down the sides as necessary.

4.Beat the egg whites: Sprinkle cream of tartar over the egg whites and whisk until they form soft peaks. Transfer about a third of the egg white mixture to the food processor and pulse until just combined. Gently fold this mixture into the remaining egg whites until fully incorporated but still light and airy. Pour the batter into the prepared loaf pan.

5.Bake the bread: Place the pan in the preheated oven and bake for approximately 30 minutes, or until the bread is golden brown and a toothpick inserted into the centre comes out clean.

6.Cool the bread: Run a thin knife around the edges of the loaf, then let it rest for 10 minutes. Turn the bread out onto a wire rack and allow it to cool completely before slicing.

Nutritional value
Carbs=19g

Calories=241
Protein=10g
Fats=21g

9.Creamy Cottage Cheese Scrambled Eggs

Prep Time:5 mins
Cook Time:5 mins
Total Time:10 mins

<u>Ingredients</u>

- 1 tablespoon butter
- 4 large eggs, beaten
- ¼ cup cottage cheese
- 1 teaspoon chopped fresh chives, or to taste (Optional)
- ground black pepper to taste

<u>Directions</u>

1. Collect all the necessary ingredients.

2. In a skillet, melt the butter over medium heat. Add the beaten eggs to the skillet and cook without stirring until the eggs start to firm up on the bottom, which should take about 1 to 2 minutes.

3. Mix in the cottage cheese and chives with the eggs, then season with black pepper.

4. Continue cooking and stirring the mixture until the eggs are almost fully set, which will take an additional 3 to 4 minutes.

Nutritional value
Carbs=2g
Calories=232
Protein=18g
Fats=19g

10.Brown Rice and Corn Cakes

Prep Time:15 mins
Cook Time:15 mins

Total Time:30 mins
Servings:7

Ingredients

- 2 (15.25 ounce) cans whole kernel sweet corn, drained
- 2 cups cooked brown rice, cooled
- ½ cup skim milk
- 2 eggs, beaten
- 2 tablespoons chopped fresh chives
- ⅔ cup whole wheat flour
- 2 teaspoons baking powder
- ⅛ teaspoon ground nutmeg
- salt and ground black pepper to taste
- 1 tablespoon olive oil, or as needed

Directions

1. In a large bowl, combine corn, rice, milk, eggs, and chives.

2. In another bowl, mix together the flour, baking powder, nutmeg, salt, and black pepper.

3. Gradually stir the flour mixture into the corn mixture until well blended.

4. Warm olive oil on a griddle or large skillet over medium heat.

5. Spoon 1/4-cup portions of the corn batter onto the heated griddle. Cook each side until golden brown, about 3 to 4 minutes per side.

<u>Nutritional value</u>
Carbs=53g
Calories=285
Protein=9g
Fat=6g

Chapter5:
Fresh and Flavorful
Lunches

1.Turkey Corn Chowder

Prep Time:20 mins
Cook Time:40 mins
Total Time:1 hr
Servings:8

Ingredients

- 3 potatoes, peeled and diced
- 2 smoked turkey legs
- ¼ cup butter
- 1 large onion, chopped
- 3 tablespoons all-purpose flour
- 1 (32 ounce) carton chicken broth
- 1 (16 ounce) package frozen corn
- 1 quart light cream

- salt and ground black pepper to taste

<u>Directions</u>

1. Place potatoes in a pot, cover with salted water, and bring to a boil. Reduce heat, cover, and simmer until tender, about 20 minutes. Drain and let them steam dry briefly. Remove meat from turkey legs, discard bones and tendons, then chop the meat and set aside.

2. In a soup pot, melt butter over medium heat. Sauté onion until translucent, about 8 minutes. Sprinkle flour over butter and onion, stirring constantly until a paste forms. Let it cook for about 1 minute. Gradually whisk in chicken broth, potatoes, turkey meat, and corn. Stir until mixture gently boils and thickens, about 5 minutes. Using a potato masher, slightly mash potatoes and vegetables until potatoes are rounded. Add cream, bring soup back to a simmer, and cook gently for 5 minutes, stirring constantly. Season with salt and pepper to taste.

<u>**Nutritional value**</u>
Carbs=41g
Calories=464
Protein=26g
Fats=28g

2.Quinoa Salad with Winter Veggies and Buffalo Chicken Sausage.

Servings:8

<u>**Ingredients**</u>

- ¾ cup uncooked quinoa
- 1 ¼ cups low-sodium chicken broth
- 3 tablespoons olive oil
- 6 links Dietz & Watson Buffalo Chicken Sausage, cut into chunks
- 1 medium onion, diced
- 2 cups butternut squash, cut into 1/2-inch cubes
- 1 cup shredded carrot
- ½ teaspoon ground cumin

- ¼ teaspoon salt
- ¼ teaspoon freshly ground black pepper
- 1 medium red bell pepper, diced
- ¼ cup fresh flat-leaf parsley, chopped

<u>Directions</u>

1. Combine quinoa and chicken broth in a saucepan. Bring to a boil, then simmer covered over low heat until liquid is absorbed, approximately 12 to 15 minutes. Fluff with a fork.

2. Meanwhile, in a large skillet over medium-high heat, heat 1 tablespoon of oil. Cook sausage, stirring occasionally, until browned, about 5 minutes. Transfer sausage to a plate.

3. Add another tablespoon of oil to the skillet. Sauté onion until softened, about 3 minutes. Add squash and carrots; cook for 5 minutes until vegetables are tender yet firm.

4. In a large bowl, whisk together lemon juice, remaining oil, cumin, salt, and pepper. Add cooked quinoa, sausage, sautéed vegetables, and onion mixture; mix well. Chill in the refrigerator for at

least 30 minutes or up to two days. Before serving, stir in parsley.

<u>Nutritional value</u>
Carbs=21g
Calories=228
Protein=17g
Fats=11g

3.Vegetable Steamed Tilapia

Prep Time:20 mins
Cook Time:20 mins
Total Time:40 mins
Servings:6

<u>Ingredients</u>
- 1 teaspoon olive oil, or as needed
- 6 tilapia fillets
- 4 stalks celery, halved lengthwise and crosswise
- 1 cup fresh baby carrots

- 1 bell pepper, cut into chunks
- ½ red onion, sliced
- 1 pinch Greek seasoning, or to taste
- salt and ground black pepper to taste

<u>Directions</u>

1. Preheat your oven to 450 degrees F (230 degrees C). Cover a baking sheet with foil and lightly brush with olive oil.

2. Place the tilapia fillets on the prepared baking sheet. Arrange celery, carrots, bell pepper, and red onion over the fillets. Season with Greek seasoning, salt, and black pepper. Cover with another sheet of foil, folding the edges to seal.

3. Bake in the preheated oven until the fish easily flakes with a fork, approximately 20 minutes.

<u>Nutritional value</u>
Carbs=6g
Calories=141g
Protein=24g
Fats=2g

4.Cucumber Sandwiches

Prep Time:15 mins
Additional Time:10 mins
Total Time:25 mins
Servings:12

<u>Ingredients</u>

- 1 cucumber, peeled and thinly sliced
- 1 (8 ounce) package cream cheese, softened
- ¼ cup mayonnaise
- ¼ teaspoon garlic powder
- ¼ teaspoon onion salt
- 1 dash Worcestershire sauce
- 1 (1 pound) loaf sliced bread, crusts removed
- 1 pinch lemon pepper (Optional

<u>Directions</u>

1. Collect all the necessary ingredients.

2. Place cucumber slices between two layers of paper towels in a colander to drain excess liquid, approximately 10 minutes.

3. Combine cream cheese, mayonnaise, garlic powder, onion salt, and Worcestershire sauce in a bowl until the mixture is smooth.
4. Evenly spread the cream cheese mixture onto one side of each slice of bread.
5. Distribute cucumber slices onto half of the bread slices; sprinkle lemon pepper over the cucumbers.
6. Place the remaining bread slices spread-side down over the cucumbers to create sandwiches; cut each sandwich into triangles.

<u>Nutritional value</u>
Carbs=25g
Calories=203
Protein=5g
Fats=11g

5.Easy Korean Beef Bowl

Prep Time:10 mins

Cook Time:15 mins
Total Time:25 mins
Servings:4

Ingredients

- 1 pound lean ground beef
- 5 cloves garlic, crushed
- 1 tablespoon freshly grated ginger
- 2 teaspoons toasted sesame oil
- ½ cup reduced-sodium soy sauce
- ⅓ cup light brown sugar
- ¼ teaspoon crushed red pepper
- 6 green onions, chopped, divided
- 4 cups hot cooked brown rice
- 1 tablespoon toasted sesame seeds

Directions

1. Heat a large skillet over medium-high heat. Add ground beef and cook, stirring and breaking into small pieces until browned, approximately 5 to 7 minutes. Remove excess grease.

2. Add minced garlic, ginger, and sesame oil to the skillet. Cook until aromatic, around 2 minutes. Mix in soy sauce, brown sugar, and red pepper flakes. Simmer until the beef absorbs some of the sauce, about 7 minutes. Stir in half of the chopped green onions.

3. Serve the beef mixture over hot cooked rice. Garnish with sesame seeds and the remaining green onions.

<u>Nutritional value</u>
Carbs=70g
Calories=575
Protein=29g
Fats=19g

6.Asian-Style Ground Beef Cabbage Wraps

Prep Time:20 mins
Cook Time:20 mins

Total Time:40 mins
Servings:4

<u>Ingredients</u>

- 1 pound lean ground beef
- 1 cup diced fresh mushrooms
- ½ cup diced onion
- 3 tablespoons coconut aminos (soy-free seasoning sauce)
- 2 teaspoons Sriracha sauce, or to taste
- 2 teaspoons minced fresh ginger
- 1 large clove garlic, minced
- 1 teaspoon rice vinegar, or to taste
- 1 teaspoon sesame oil
- salt and ground black pepper to taste
- 8 leaves cabbage
- ½ cup matchstick-cut carrots
- 3 green onions, thinly sliced
- 8 sprigs cilantro, or to taste (Optional)
- 1 pinch sesame seeds (Optional)
- 1 pinch red pepper flakes (Optional)

Directions

1. Heat a large skillet over medium-high heat. Cook ground beef until browned and crumbly, about 5 minutes. Add mushrooms and onion; cook and stir until vegetables soften, about 4 minutes.
2. Stir in coconut aminos, Sriracha sauce, ginger, garlic, and vinegar. Cook, stirring occasionally, until most of the liquid evaporates, about 10 minutes. Remove from heat and mix in sesame oil. Season with salt and pepper.
3. Spoon the mixture evenly onto 8 cabbage leaves. Sprinkle it with carrots, green onions, cilantro, sesame seeds, and red pepper flakes. Roll each cabbage leaf around the filling to form a packet.

Nutritional value
Carbs=13g
Calories=285
Protein=22g
Fats=18g

7. Creamy Roasted Parsnip Soup

Prep Time:30 mins
Cook Time:50 mins
Total Time:1 hr 20 mins
Servings:10

<u>Ingredients</u>

- 2 pounds parsnips, peeled and cut into 1/2 inch pieces
- 3 carrots, peeled and cut into 1/2-inch pieces
- 2 tablespoons olive oil, divided
- sea salt and ground black pepper to taste
- 1 large onion, diced
- 3 stalks celery, diced
- 1 tablespoon butter
- 1 tablespoon brown sugar
- 3 cloves garlic, minced
- 1 teaspoon ground ginger
- ½ teaspoon ground cardamom
- ½ teaspoon ground allspice
- ½ teaspoon ground nutmeg
- ¼ teaspoon cayenne pepper
- 4 cups chicken stock

- 1 cup whole milk
- ½ cup heavy cream

<u>Directions</u>

1. Preheat your oven to 425 degrees F (220 degrees C).

2. Place parsnips and carrots in a bowl, drizzle with 1 tablespoon of olive oil, and toss well to coat. Season with salt and pepper. Spread the vegetables evenly on a baking sheet.

3. Roast in the preheated oven until the vegetables are tender and the parsnips are golden brown, approximately 30 minutes.

4. In a large saucepan over medium heat, heat the remaining 1 tablespoon of olive oil. Cook and stir the onion and celery until softened and the onion starts to turn golden brown, about 5 minutes. Reduce the heat to low. Add butter, brown sugar, garlic, and the roasted parsnips and carrots. Continue to cook and stir until the vegetables are very soft and beginning to brown, about 5 to 10 minutes.

5. Working in batches, transfer the soup to a blender, filling it no more than halfway. Securely

hold down the blender lid with a folded kitchen towel and carefully pulse a few times to start blending before puréeing until smooth. Pour the blended soup back into a clean pot.

6. Stir in the milk and cream. Return to a simmer over medium-low heat. Season with salt and pepper to taste before serving.

<u>Nutritional value</u>
Carbs=187
Calories=187
Protein=3g
Fats=10g

8.Sesame Seared Tuna and Sushi Bar Spinach Salad

Prep Time:15 mins
Cook Time:5 mins
Total Time:20 mins
Servings:2

Ingredients

For the Spinach Salad:
- ½ pound baby spinach leaves
- 3 tablespoons white sesame seeds
- 1 tablespoon white sugar
- 1 tablespoon soy sauce, or to taste
- ½ teaspoon mirin

For the Miso Mayo Sauce:
- ¼ cup mayonnaise
- 2 teaspoons white miso paste
- 1 tablespoon seasoned rice vinegar

For the Seared Tuna:
- 2 (5 ounce) sushi-grade ahi tuna steaks
- salt to taste
- 2 tablespoons black sesame seeds
- 2 teaspoons vegetable oil
- 1 tablespoon prepared ponzu sauce

Directions

1. Heat spinach in a dry pot over medium-high heat until it just starts to wilt, about 1 to 2 minutes. Transfer to a strainer to cool.
2. While the spinach cools, toast white sesame seeds in a dry pan over medium heat until lightly golden. Crush them coarsely in a mortar and pestle, leaving some seeds whole. Mix with white sugar, soy sauce, and mirin using a wooden spoon. Set aside.
3. Squeeze any excess liquid from the cooled spinach using a towel. Chop roughly and place in a mixing bowl. Add the prepared dressing and mix well. Cover and refrigerate until thoroughly chilled before serving.
4. Prepare the miso mayo sauce by combining mayonnaise, miso paste, and rice vinegar. Chill in the refrigerator until ready to use.
5. Lightly salt the tuna steaks, then coat all sides generously with sesame seeds, pressing lightly.
6. Brush a nonstick pan with oil and heat over medium heat. Sear the tuna steaks for 30 to 45 seconds on each side and each edge.

7. Slice the tuna and serve over the miso sauce. Brush with ponzu and serve alongside the spinach salad.

Nutritional value
Carbs=20g
Calories=597
Protein=43g
Fat=40g

9.Baked Potato Soup

Prep Time:15 mins
Cook Time:25 mins
Total Time:40 mins
Servings:6

Ingredients
- 12 slices bacon

- ⅔ cup butter
- ⅔ cup all-purpose flour
- 7 cups milk
- 4 large baked potatoes, peeled and cubed
- 4 green onions, chopped
- 1 ¼ cups shredded Cheddar cheese
- 1 cup sour cream
- 1 teaspoon salt
- 1 teaspoon ground black pepper

Directions

1. Prepare all ingredients.

2. Cook bacon in a large skillet on medium-high heat until evenly browned, about 8 to 10 minutes. Drain on paper towels, crumble, and set aside.

3. In a stockpot or Dutch oven, melt butter over medium heat. Gradually add flour, whisking until smooth. Slowly pour in milk, whisking constantly until the mixture is thick and smooth.

4. Add potatoes and onions, bring to a boil, and stir frequently. Reduce heat and simmer for 10 minutes.

5. Stir in crumbled bacon, Cheddar cheese, sour cream, salt, and pepper. Continue to cook and stir until the cheese is melted.

6. Serve and enjoy!

Nutritional value

Carbs=50g
Calories=745
Protein=27g
Fats=49g

10. Pesto Spaghetti Frittata

Prep Time:10 mins
Cook Time:35 mins
Total Time:45 mins
Servings:5

Ingredients

- 6 duck eggs
- 1/2 cup shredded Parmesan cheese
- 1/4 cup half-and-half cream
- 1/4 cup ricotta cheese

- 2 tablespoons prepared pesto, plus more for garnish
- 1 teaspoon fresh thyme leaves
- 1/2 teaspoon salt
- 1/4 teaspoon freshly ground black pepper
- 1 pound frozen mixed carrots, broccoli, zucchini, and cauliflower 1 tablespoon unsalted butter
- 2 cloves garlic, minced
- 4 ounces leftover cooked spaghetti pasta

Directions

1. Preheat your oven to 400 degrees F (200 degrees C).

2. In a large bowl, combine eggs, Parmesan cheese, half and half, ricotta, pesto, thyme, salt, and pepper, and whisk until smooth.

3. Place the vegetables in a microwave-safe bowl and microwave on High until thawed, about 4 to 5 minutes. Drain well.

4. In an ovenproof nonstick skillet, melt butter over medium heat. Add garlic and cook until fragrant,

approximately 1 minute. Add the steamed vegetables and toss to coat.

5. Pour half of the egg mixture into the skillet. Toss the cooked spaghetti with the remaining egg mixture, then pour the egg-coated pasta into the skillet. Cook for 5 minutes.

6. Transfer the skillet to the preheated oven and bake until the eggs are set, about 25 minutes. Remove from the oven, cut into wedges, and serve with additional pesto if desired.

Nutritional value
Carbs=16g
Calories=244
Protein=12g
Fat=13g

Chapter6: Satisfying Dinners for Every Occasion

1.Green Bean and Mushroom Medley

Prep Time:20 mins
Cook Time:15 mins
Total Time:35 mins
Servings:6

Ingredients

- ½ pound fresh green beans, cut into 1-inch lengths
- 2 carrots, cut into thick strips
- ¼ cup butter
- 1 onion, sliced
- ½ pound fresh mushrooms, sliced
- 1 teaspoon salt

- ½ teaspoon seasoned salt
- ¼ teaspoon garlic salt
- ¼ teaspoon white pepper

<u>Directions</u>

1. Fill a pot with 1 inch of water and bring it to a boil over high heat. Add green beans and carrots to the boiling water. Cover and cook until they are tender but still slightly firm. Then, drain them.

2. In a large skillet, melt butter over medium heat. Cook onions and mushrooms until they are nearly tender. Lower the heat, cover the skillet, and let it simmer for 3 minutes.

3. Add the cooked green beans and carrots to the skillet. Season with salt, seasoned salt, garlic salt, and white pepper. Cover and cook over medium heat for 5 minutes.

<u>Nutritional value</u>
Carbs=11g
Calories=109

Protein=3g
Fat=7g

2.Chicken, Broccoli, and Cheddar Casserole

Prep Time:20 mins
Cook Time:30 mins
Total Time:50 mins
Servings:8

<u>Ingredients</u>

- 3 cups cooked shredded chicken
- 2 cups cooked chopped broccoli
- 2 (10.5 ounce) cans condensed cream of chicken soup
- 1/2 cup sour cream
- 1 pinch ground black pepper to taste
- 2 1/2 cups shredded Cheddar cheese
- 1 1/2 cups bread crumbs
- 1/4 cup salted butter, melted

Directions

1. Preheat your oven to 375 degrees Fahrenheit (190 degrees Celsius).

2. In a bowl, mix together chicken, broccoli, condensed soup, sour cream, pepper, and 1 cup of Cheddar cheese. Transfer the mixture into a 2-quart casserole dish and sprinkle the remaining Cheddar cheese on top.

3. Combine bread crumbs and melted butter in another bowl, then sprinkle this mixture evenly over the casserole.

4. Bake in the preheated oven until the casserole is bubbly and the cheese is fully melted, which typically takes about 30 to 35 minutes.

Nutritional value

Carbs=19g
Calories=475
Protein=32g
Fats=28g

3.Classic Beef Stuffed Peppers

Prep Time:20 mins
Cook Time:1 hr
Total Time:1 hr 20 mins
Servings:5

Ingredients

- 6 red bell peppers - tops and seeds removed
- 3 eggs, beaten
- 3 cups meatless spaghetti sauce
- 1 ¼ cups instant rice
- ¼ cup finely chopped onion
- 1 teaspoon salt
- 1 ½ teaspoons Worcestershire sauce
- 1 pinch ground black pepper
- 1 ½ pounds lean ground beef
- 2 cups meatless spaghetti sauce
- 6 tablespoons shredded Cheddar cheese divided

Directions

1. Preheat your oven to 350°F (175°C).

2. Boil the red bell peppers until slightly softened, about 5 minutes, then drain and rinse them with cold water.

3. In a bowl, mix together eggs, 3 cups of spaghetti sauce, instant rice, onion, salt, Worcestershire sauce, and black pepper. Add crumbled ground beef and combine thoroughly.

4. Stand the peppers upright in a large baking dish and fill each pepper with the beef mixture. Pour 2 cups of spaghetti sauce over the peppers. Cover the dish with aluminium foil.

5. Bake in the preheated oven for 55 to 60 minutes, until the peppers are tender and the filling is set. Ensure the internal temperature reaches at least 160°F (70°C).

6. Uncover the dish and sprinkle 1 tablespoon of Cheddar cheese on top of each pepper. Let it melt slightly before serving.

<u>Nutritional value</u>
Carbs=57g

Calories=604
Protein=35g
Fats=28g

4.Roasted Sweet Potato and Kale Salad.

Prep Time:20 mins
Cook Time:20 mins
Additional Time:35 mins
Total Time:1 hr 15 mins
Servings:6

<u>Ingredients</u>

- 2 sweet potatoes or jewel yams, cut into 1-inch cubes
- 2 tablespoons olive oil
- salt and freshly ground black pepper to taste
- 1 tablespoon olive oil
- 1 onion, sliced
- 3 cloves garlic, minced
- 1 bunch kale, torn into bite-sized pieces

- 2 tablespoons red wine vinegar
- 1 teaspoon chopped fresh thyme

<u>Directions</u>

1. Preheat your oven to 400 degrees F (200 degrees C). Toss sweet potato cubes with 2 tablespoons of olive oil in a bowl. Season with salt and pepper to taste, then spread evenly on a baking sheet.

2. Bake in the preheated oven until the sweet potatoes are tender, about 20 to 25 minutes. Let them cool to room temperature in the refrigerator.

3. Meanwhile, in a large skillet over medium heat, heat the remaining 1 tablespoon of olive oil. Add onion and garlic, cooking and stirring until the onion caramelised to a golden brown, approximately 15 minutes. Add kale and cook until it wilts and becomes tender. Transfer the kale mixture to a bowl and let it cool to room temperature in the refrigerator.

4. Once all the components are cooled, combine the sweet potatoes, kale, red wine vinegar, and fresh thyme in a bowl. Season with salt and pepper to taste, gently stirring to mix everything together.

Nutritional value
Carbs=49g
Calories=285
Protein=7g
Fats=9g

5.Savory Roasted Root Vegetables.

Prep Time:30 mins
Cook Time:45 mins
Total Time:1 hr 15 mins
Servings:6

Ingredients
- 1 cup diced, raw beet
- 4 carrots, diced
- 1 onion, diced
- 2 cups diced potatoes
- 4 cloves garlic, minced
- ¼ cup canned garbanzo beans (chickpeas), drained

- 2 tablespoons olive oil
- 1 tablespoon dried thyme leaves
- salt and pepper to taste
- ⅓ cup dry white wine
- 1 cup torn beet greens

Directions

1. Preheat your oven to 400 degrees F (200 degrees C).

2. In a 9x13 inch baking dish, combine beets, carrots, onions, potatoes, garlic, and chickpeas. Drizzle with olive oil and season with thyme, salt, and pepper. Mix thoroughly.

3. Bake uncovered in the preheated oven for 30 minutes, stirring halfway through. Remove from the oven, add wine, and bake for an additional 15 minutes until most of the wine evaporates and the vegetables are tender. Stir in beet greens to wilt them. Season with salt and pepper to taste before serving.

Nutritional value

Carbs=21g
Calories=147
Protein=4g
Fat=4g

6.Roast Duck Legs With Red Wine Sauce.

Prep Time:5 mins
Cook Time:1 hr 15 mins
Total Time:1 hr 20 mins
Servings:8

Ingredients

- 1 bunch chopped fresh rosemary
- 4 large garlic cloves
- 4 duck legs
- salt to taste
- 1 teaspoon Chinese five-spice powder
- 1 ½ cups red wine

- 1 ½ tablespoons red currant jelly

Directions

1. Preheat your oven to 375 degrees F (190 degrees C). Spread out rosemary sprigs and garlic cloves in a 9x13-inch baking dish.

2. Arrange the duck legs on top of the rosemary, season with salt and five-spice powder. Bake in the preheated oven for 1 hour. Meanwhile, in a small saucepan, bring the wine to a boil over medium-high heat. Stir in the currant jelly until dissolved. Reduce heat to medium-low and simmer for 5 minutes; then set aside.

3. After baking the duck for 1 hour, remove and discard any accumulated fat from the baking dish. Pour the wine sauce over the duck legs and bake for an additional 15 minutes, or until the duck is very tender and the sauce has slightly thickened.

Nutritional value

Carbs=14g
Calories=244
Protein=16g
Fat=8g

7.Grilled Tofu Skewers with Sriracha Sauce

Prep Time:15 mins
Cook Time:10 mins
Additional Time:1 hr
Total Time:1 hr 25 mins
Serving:2

<u>Ingredients</u>

- 1 (8 ounce) container extra firm tofu, drained and sliced into large chunks
- 1 zucchini, cut into large chunks
- 1 red bell pepper, cut into large chunks
- 10 large mushrooms

- 2 tablespoons sriracha chilli garlic sauce
- ¼ cup soy sauce
- 2 tablespoons sesame oil
- ¼ cup diced onion
- 1 jalapeno pepper, diced
- ground black pepper to taste

Directions

1. Combine tofu, zucchini, red bell pepper, and mushrooms in a bowl. In a separate small bowl, mix sriracha sauce, soy sauce, sesame oil, onion, jalapeno, and pepper. Pour this mixture over the tofu and vegetables, tossing gently to coat. Cover and marinate in the refrigerator for at least 1 hour.

2. Preheat an outdoor grill to medium-high heat and lightly oil the grate.

3. Thread the marinated tofu and vegetables onto skewers. Grill each skewer for about 10 minutes or until cooked to your liking. Serve with any remaining marinade as a dipping sauce.

Nutritional value

Carbs=22g
Calories=312
Protein=15g
Fat=21g

8.Spicy Tan Tan Soup (Tantanmen or Dan Dan Noodles)

Prep Time:10 mins
Cook Time:15 mins
Total Time:25 mins
Servings:2

Ingredients

- 1 teaspoon sesame oil
- 2 teaspoons doubanjiang (soy bean paste)
- 1 tablespoon minced shallots
- 1 clove garlic, pressed
- 1 ½ teaspoons grated fresh ginger
- 6 ounces ground pork
- ¼ cup soy sauce
- 2 tablespoons tahini (sesame seed paste)
- 1 tablespoon sake

- 1 tablespoon miso paste
- 1 teaspoon tianmianjiang (sweet bean paste)
- 4 cups chicken stock
- 2 teaspoons rice vinegar
- 1 teaspoon rayu (chile oil)
- ½ cup fresh spinach, or to taste (Optional)
- 2 cups ramen noodles, or to taste
- 3 green onions, thinly sliced
- 1 red Thai chile pepper, sliced

Directions

1. Heat sesame oil in a skillet over medium heat. Add doubanjiang and stir in shallots, garlic, and ginger until fragrant, about 30 seconds. Add ground pork and cook until browned, approximately 3 minutes.

2. Combine soy sauce, tahini, sake, miso paste, and tianmianjiang with the pork mixture until well blended. Pour in chicken stock and bring to a boil. Stir in rice vinegar and rayu, then add spinach. Let the soup simmer over low heat for 10 minutes.

3. Place noodles in hot water to separate and drain. Stir noodles into the soup and garnish with green onions and Thai chili peppers.

Nutritional value
Carbs=41g
Calories=564
Protein=32g
Fat=32g

9.Oven-Baked Potato Fries

Prep Time:10 mins
Cook Time:30 mins
Total Time:40 mins
Servings:5

Ingredients
- 2 pounds baking potatoes, each cut into six wedges
- 2 tablespoons olive oil
- ½ teaspoon dried thyme leaves
- ¼ teaspoon ground black pepper
- salt to taste

- ¼ cup shredded Cheddar cheese (Optional)

Directions

1. Gather all your ingredients and preheat the oven to 450°F (230°C).
2. Place the potato wedges on a baking sheet. Drizzle them with olive oil and season with thyme, pepper, and salt. Use a spatula to toss the wedges, ensuring they're evenly coated.
3. Roast the potato wedges in the preheated oven for 15 minutes. Then, flip them over and roast for another 15 minutes or until they are soft in the middle.
4. Transfer the roasted wedges to a serving platter and sprinkle with cheese before serving.

Nutritional value
Carbs=45g
Calories=265
Protein=4g
Fats=8g

10.Hawaiian Beef Teriyaki Stir-Fry Bowl

Prep Time:20 mins
Cook Time:25 mins
Additional Time:45 mins
Total Time:1 hr 30 mins
Servings:4

<u>Ingredients</u>

- 1 cup water
- ¼ cup pineapple juice
- 5 tablespoons brown sugar
- 1 tablespoon tamari
- 1 clove garlic, grated
- ½ teaspoon ginger paste
- ⅛ teaspoon onion powder
- 1 tablespoon tapioca flour
- 1 (8 ounce) thinly sliced carne asada (beef steak)
- 1 tablespoon grapeseed oil

- 1 pinch red pepper flakes
- 1 red bell pepper, cut into strips
- 1 green bell pepper, cut into strips
- 1 small yellow onion, quartered and sliced
- 2 carrots, sliced diagonally
- 14 ounces refrigerated chow mein noodles
- 1 teaspoon everything bagel seasoning
- 1 tablespoon chopped green onion, or to taste

Directions

1. Combine water, pineapple juice, brown sugar, tamari, garlic, ginger paste, and onion powder in a zip-top bag. Set aside 1/2 cup of this mixture and mix it with tapioca flour. Cut the beef into 1-inch pieces, add to the bag, seal, and refrigerate for 45 minutes.

2. Heat oil in a multi-functional pressure cooker using the Saute function. Add red pepper flakes and beef pieces (discard marinade). Cook until browned, about 5 to 7 minutes.

3. Place bell peppers, onions, and carrots in a steamer basket above the meat. Cancel the Saute function.

4. Close and lock the lid. Set the pressure cooker to high pressure for 3 minutes. Allow pressure to build for 10 to 15 minutes.

5. Release pressure using the quick-release method (about 5 minutes). Unlock and remove the lid. Carefully take out the steamer basket with vegetables and set aside.

6. Switch back to Saute mode, add noodles to the pressure cooker. Stir in the reserved marinade mixed with tapioca until the sauce thickens. Add back the cooked vegetables. Toss everything together.

7. Serve immediately in bowls, garnished with everything bagel seasoning and green onions.

Nutritional value
Carbs=85g
Calories=744
Protein=20g
Fats=35g

Chapter7:
Irresistible Snacks, Plant Based and Desserts.

1.Creamy Rice Pudding

Prep Time:10 mins
Cook Time:40 mins
Total Time:50 mins
Servings:6

Ingredients

- 1 ½ cups cold water
- ¾ cup uncooked white rice
- 2 cups milk, divided
- ⅓ cup white sugar
- ¼ teaspoon salt
- 1 large egg, beaten
- ⅔ cup golden raisins
- 1 tablespoon butter
- ½ teaspoon vanilla extract

Directions

1. Start by bringing water to a boil in a saucepan. Add rice, reduce heat to low, cover, and simmer until rice is tender and the liquid is absorbed, approximately 20 minutes.

2. Transfer the cooked rice to another saucepan. Add 1 ½ cups of milk, sugar, and salt. Cook over medium heat, stirring frequently, until the mixture thickens and becomes creamy, about 15 minutes.

3. Stir in the remaining 1/2 cup of milk, beaten egg, and raisins. Cook for an additional 2 minutes, stirring constantly. Remove from heat and mix in butter and vanilla until well combined. Serve the dish warm.

Nutritional value
Carbs=74g
Calories=370
Protein=9g
Fats=7g

2.Pecan Pie Energy Bites

Prep Time:15 mins
Cook Time:10 mins
Total Time:25 mins
Servings:12

Ingredients

- 1 cup pecan halves
- ⅓ cup rolled oats
- 1 cup pitted Medjool dates
- ⅛ teaspoon ground cinnamon
- ¼ teaspoon kosher salt
- ¼ teaspoon vanilla extract
- 1 tablespoon maple syrup

Directions

1. Preheat your oven to 350 degrees F (175 degrees C) and line a baking sheet with parchment paper.

2. Spread pecans in a single layer on the prepared baking sheet and add rolled oats on top. Bake in the preheated oven for about 10 minutes until toasted. Let them cool completely.

3. In a food processor, pulse together the toasted pecans, oats, dates, cinnamon, salt, vanilla extract, and maple syrup until the nuts are ground to your desired texture.

4. Form the mixture into twelve tightly-packed 2-inch balls. Chill in the refrigerator before serving.

Nutritional value
Carbs=18g
Calories=117
Protein=4g
Fats=8g

3. Granola Bars

Prep Time:15 mins
Cook Time:25 mins
Additional Time:1 hr
Total Time:1 hr 40 mins
Servings:8

Ingredients

- cooking spray
- 2 cups rolled oats
- ½ cup shredded coconut
- ½ cup honey
- 2 tablespoons creamy peanut butter
- 1 teaspoon vanilla extract
- ⅛ teaspoon salt

Directions

1. Gather all the ingredients. Preheat your oven to 325 degrees F (165 degrees C) and grease a 9-inch square baking dish.

2. Spread oats and coconut evenly on a baking sheet. Toast them in the preheated oven until they turn brown, which takes about 10 minutes. Then, transfer them to a large mixing bowl.

3. In a saucepan over medium-low heat, combine honey, peanut butter, vanilla extract, and salt. Stir the mixture until it becomes smooth and well combined.

4. Pour the honey mixture over the oats and coconut in the mixing bowl. Stir thoroughly to coat everything evenly. Then, spread this mixture evenly into the prepared baking dish.

5. Bake in the preheated oven until the granola bars begin to dry out, approximately 15 minutes for crunchy bars or less time if you prefer them chewy.

6. Allow the bars to cool completely in the baking dish before cutting them into desired shapes and sizes.

Nutritional value
Carbs=34g
Calories=188
Protein=4g
Fat=5g

4.Pina Colada Sorbet

Prep Time:25 mins
Total Time:25 mins
Serving:8

Ingredients

- 1 ½ cups white sugar
- 1 ½ cups water
- 1 (20 ounce) can canned crushed pineapple, drained
- 1 (13.5 ounce) can coconut milk
- ¼ cup lime juice

Directions

1. Create a syrup by boiling sugar and water in a small saucepan over high heat until the liquid turns clear, approximately 1 minute. Let it cool.

2. Blend the drained pineapple in a blender or food processor until it's smooth and frothy. In a large bowl, combine the syrup, pineapple puree, coconut milk, and lime juice. Chill in the refrigerator for about 3 hours.

3. Freeze the mixture in an ice cream maker according to the manufacturer's instructions.

Nutritional value
Carbs=55g
Calories=295
Protein=2g
Fat=10g

5.Banana Split Chia Seed Pudding

Prep Time:10 mins
Refrigerated Time:4 hrs
Total Time:4 hrs 10 mins
Servings:4

Ingredients

- 1 cup Almond Breeze Unsweetened Vanilla Almond Milk
- 1/2 cup plain Greek yoghourts
- 1 1/2 tablespoons pure maple syrup
- 1/2 teaspoon vanilla extract
- 1/4 cup chia seeds
- 1 banana, thinly sliced

- 1/2 cup chopped strawberries
- 1/2 cup blueberries
- 1/4 cup unsweetened coconut flakes, toasted
- 2 tablespoons cacao nibs

Directions

1. Combine Almond Breeze Unsweetened Vanilla Almond Milk, Greek yoghurt, maple syrup, and vanilla in a container. Mix in chia seeds, cover, and refrigerate for at least 4 hours or overnight.

2. When ready to serve, toast coconut flakes in a sauté pan over medium heat until golden (1-3 minutes). Remove from heat and let cool.

3. Stir chia seed pudding to remove any lumps. Divide into 4 serving dishes and top with sliced bananas, strawberries, blueberries, toasted coconut flakes, and cacao nibs evenly.

Nutritional value

Carbs=25g
Calories=213
Protein=7g
Fat=15g

6. Cauliflower Fried 'Rice'

Prep Time:15 mins
Cook Time:30 mins
Total Time:45 mins
Servings:6

<u>Ingredients</u>

- 2 cups frozen peas
- ½ cup water
- ¼ cup sesame oil, divided
- 4 cups cubed pork loin
- 6 green onions, sliced
- 1 large carrot, cubed
- 2 cloves garlic, minced
- 20 ounces shredded cauliflower
- 6 tablespoons soy sauce
- 2 eggs, beaten

<u>Directions</u>

1. Combine peas and water in a saucepan. Bring to a boil, then simmer until peas are tender, about 5 minutes. Drain and set aside.

2. Heat 2 tablespoons of sesame oil in a wok over medium-high heat. Cook pork until browned and fully cooked, about 7 to 10 minutes. Transfer pork to a plate.

3. Add the remaining 2 tablespoons of sesame oil to the wok. Sauté green onions, carrot, and garlic until softened, about 5 minutes. Add cauliflower and cook until tender but still firm, about 4 to 5 minutes.

4. Return pork and peas to the wok. Stir in soy sauce and stir-fry until heated through and slightly browned, about 3 to 5 minutes.

5. Push the pork mixture to one side of the wok. Pour beaten eggs into the empty space and scramble until cooked through, about 3 to 5 minutes. Stir the cooked eggs into the pork mixture, breaking up any large pieces.

<u>Nutritional value</u>
Carbs=19g

**Calories=368
Protein=45g
Fats=19g**

BONUS PAGE.

BONUS 1:30-Day Meal Plan.

Day 1
Breakfast: Rice porridge with coconut milk and a sprinkle of cinnamon
Lunch: Grilled turkey breast with steamed zucchini and white rice
Dinner: Baked cod with mashed potatoes and green beans
Snack: Pear slices

Day 2
Breakfast: Oatmeal with blueberries and a drizzle of honey
Lunch: Chicken salad with iceberg lettuce, cucumber, and a squeeze of lemon
Dinner: Beef stir-fry with bok choy and jasmine rice
Snack: Plain yoghourt with a few drops of maple syrup

Day 3
Breakfast: Buckwheat pancakes with a side of apple slices
Lunch: Turkey and cheese sandwich on white bread with a side of steamed carrots
Dinner: Lamb chops with mashed parsnips and sautéed green beans
Snack: Rice cakes with a spread of cottage cheese

Day 4
Breakfast: Smoothie with banana, almond milk, and a dash of vanilla
Lunch: Lentil soup with a side of gluten-free crackers
Dinner: Baked chicken thighs with quinoa and roasted Brussels sprouts
Snack: Sliced pear with a handful of sunflower seeds

Day 5
Breakfast: Millet porridge with a handful of blueberries
Lunch: Tuna salad with iceberg lettuce, cucumber, and olive oil dressing

Dinner: Pork tenderloin with steamed broccoli and sweet potato mash

Snack: Plain rice cakes with a slice of cheese

Day 6

Breakfast: Quinoa porridge with a drizzle of maple syrup and a sprinkle of coconut flakes

Lunch: Chicken wrap with lettuce, cucumber, and dairy-free mayo in a gluten-free wrap

Dinner: Grilled salmon with asparagus and basmati rice

Snack: Fresh pear slices

Day 7

Breakfast: Rice flakes cereal with coconut milk and fresh berries

Lunch: Turkey burger with a gluten-free bun, lettuce, and avocado slices

Dinner: Baked cod with mashed potatoes and steamed green beans

Snack: Smoothie with almond milk, banana, and a dash of cinnamon

Day 8

Breakfast: Buckwheat waffles with a side of plain yoghourt and honey

Lunch: Grilled chicken breast with quinoa salad and roasted zucchini

Dinner: Beef stew with potatoes, carrots, and celery

Snack: Rice cakes with a spread of sunflower seed butter

Day 9

Breakfast: Oatmeal with fresh blueberries and a sprinkle of flax seeds

Lunch: Turkey and lettuce wrap with cucumber and dairy-free mayo

Dinner: Lamb kebabs with rice pilaf and sautéed spinach

Snack: Apple slices with a handful of pumpkin seeds

Day 10

*Breakfast:*Millet porridge with a dash of cinnamon and a drizzle of honey

Lunch: Lentil salad with diced cucumbers, tomatoes, and lemon juice

Dinner: Baked chicken thighs with roasted sweet potatoes and green beans
Snack: Plain yoghourt with a few drops of vanilla extract

Day 11
Breakfast: Smoothie with banana, almond milk, and a scoop of protein powder
Lunch: Beef stir-fry with bok choy and jasmine rice
Dinner: Grilled pork chops with mashed parsnips and steamed broccoli
Snack: Sliced pear with a few almonds

Day 12
Breakfast: Rice porridge with coconut milk and blueberries
Lunch: Turkey salad with iceberg lettuce, cucumber, and olive oil dressing
Dinner: Salmon fillet with asparagus and quinoa
Snack: Plain rice cakes with a spread of cottage cheese

Day 13

Breakfast: Buckwheat pancakes with a side of fresh fruit

Lunch: Chicken soup with carrots, celery, and gluten-free noodles

Dinner: Beef and vegetable skewers with jasmine rice

Snack: Fresh pear slices with sunflower seeds

Day 14

Breakfast: Quinoa porridge with a drizzle of maple syrup and a sprinkle of coconut flakes

Lunch: Grilled chicken breast with steamed broccoli and mashed sweet potatoes

Dinner: Lamb stew with potatoes, carrots, and celery

Snack: Plain yoghourt with a drizzle of honey

Day 15

Breakfast: Millet porridge with a handful of blueberries

Lunch: Tuna salad with iceberg lettuce, cucumber, and lemon juice

Dinner: Baked cod with roasted zucchini and basmati rice

Snack: Rice cakes with a spread of sunflower seed butter

Day 16

Breakfast: Rice flakes cereal with coconut milk and fresh berries

Lunch: Turkey burger on a gluten-free bun with lettuce and avocado slices

Dinner: Grilled salmon with steamed green beans and quinoa

Snack: Smoothie with almond milk, banana, and a dash of vanilla

Day 17

Breakfast: Buckwheat waffles with a side of plain yoghourt and honey

Lunch: Chicken wrap with lettuce, cucumber, and dairy-free mayo in a gluten-free wrap

Dinner: Beef stew with potatoes, carrots, and celery

Snack: Fresh pear slices

Day 18

Breakfast: Oatmeal with fresh blueberries and a sprinkle of flax seeds
Lunch: Turkey and lettuce wrap with cucumber and dairy-free mayo
Dinner: Pork tenderloin with steamed broccoli and sweet potato mash
Snack: Apple slices with a handful of pumpkin seeds

Day 19
Breakfast: Millet porridge with a dash of cinnamon and a drizzle of honey
Lunch: Lentil salad with diced cucumbers, tomatoes, and lemon juice
Dinner: Baked chicken thighs with roasted sweet potatoes and green beans
Snack: Plain yoghourt with a few drops of vanilla extract

Day 20
Breakfast: Smoothie with banana, almond milk, and a scoop of protein powder
Lunch: Beef stir-fry with bok choy and jasmine rice

Dinner: Grilled pork chops with mashed parsnips and steamed broccoli

Snack: Sliced pear with a few almonds

Day 21

Breakfast: Rice porridge with coconut milk and blueberries

Lunch: Turkey salad with iceberg lettuce, cucumber, and olive oil dressing

Dinner: Salmon fillet with asparagus and quinoa

Snack: Plain rice cakes with a spread of cottage cheese

Day 22

Breakfast: Buckwheat pancakes with a side of fresh fruit

Lunch: Chicken soup with carrots, celery, and gluten-free noodles

Dinner: Beef and vegetable skewers with jasmine rice

Snack: Fresh pear slices with sunflower seeds

Day 23

Breakfast: Quinoa porridge with a drizzle of maple syrup and a sprinkle of coconut flakes

Lunch: Grilled chicken breast with steamed broccoli and mashed sweet potatoes

Dinner: Lamb stew with potatoes, carrots, and celery

Snack: Plain yoghourt with a drizzle of honey

Day 24

Breakfast: Millet porridge with a handful of blueberries

Lunch: Tuna salad with iceberg lettuce, cucumber, and lemon juice

Dinner: Baked cod with roasted zucchini and basmati rice

Snack: Rice cakes with a spread of sunflower seed butter

Day 25

Breakfast: Rice flakes cereal with coconut milk and fresh berries

Lunch: Turkey burger on a gluten-free bun with lettuce and avocado slices

Dinner: Grilled salmon with steamed green beans and quinoa

Snack: Smoothie with almond milk, banana, and a dash of vanilla

Day 26

Breakfast: Buckwheat waffles with a side of plain yoghourt and honey

Lunch: Chicken wrap with lettuce, cucumber, and dairy-free mayo in a gluten-free wrap

Dinner: Beef stew with potatoes, carrots, and celery

Snack: Fresh pear slices

Day 27

Breakfast: Oatmeal with fresh blueberries and a sprinkle of flax seeds

Lunch: Turkey and lettuce wrap with cucumber and dairy-free mayo

Dinner: Pork tenderloin with steamed broccoli and sweet potato mash

Snack: Apple slices with a handful of pumpkin seeds

Day 28
Breakfast: Millet porridge with a dash of cinnamon and a drizzle of honey
Lunch: Lentil salad with diced cucumbers, tomatoes, and lemon juice
Dinner: Baked chicken thighs with roasted sweet potatoes and green beans
Snack: Plain yoghourt with a few drops of vanilla extract

Day 29
Breakfast: Smoothie with banana, almond milk, and a scoop of protein powder
Lunch: Beef stir-fry with bok choy and jasmine rice
Dinner: Grilled pork chops with mashed parsnips and steamed broccoli
Snack: Sliced pear with a few almonds

Day 30

Breakfast: Rice porridge with coconut milk and blueberries
Lunch: Turkey salad with iceberg lettuce, cucumber, and olive oil dressing

Dinner: Salmon fillet with asparagus and quinoa

Snack: Plain rice cakes with a spread of cottage cheese

BONUS   2:5 WEEKS MEAL PLAN JOURNAL.

WEEKLY MEAL PLAN JOURNAL

WEEK OF: _________

SUN	BREAKFAST:	DINNER:
	LUNCH:	SNACK:
MON	BREAKFAST:	DINNER:
	LUNCH:	SNACK:
TUE	BREAKFAST:	DINNER:
	LUNCH:	SNACK:
WED	BREAKFAST:	DINNER:
	LUNCH:	SNACK:
THU	BREAKFAST:	DINNER:
	LUNCH:	SNACK:
FRI	BREAKFAST:	DINNER:
	LUNCH:	SNACK:
SAT	BREAKFAST:	DINNER:
	LUNCH:	SNACK:

WEEKLY MEAL PLAN JOURNAL

WEEK OF: _________

SUN	BREAKFAST:	DINNER:
	LUNCH:	SNACK:
MON	BREAKFAST:	DINNER:
	LUNCH:	SNACK:
TUE	BREAKFAST:	DINNER:
	LUNCH:	SNACK:
WED	BREAKFAST:	DINNER:
	LUNCH:	SNACK:
THU	BREAKFAST:	DINNER:
	LUNCH:	SNACK:
FRI	BREAKFAST:	DINNER:
	LUNCH:	SNACK:
SAT	BREAKFAST:	DINNER:
	LUNCH:	SNACK:

WEEKLY MEAL PLAN JOURNAL

WEEK OF: _____________

SUN	BREAKFAST:	DINNER:
	LUNCH:	SNACK:
MON	BREAKFAST:	DINNER:
	LUNCH:	SNACK:
TUE	BREAKFAST:	DINNER:
	LUNCH:	SNACK:
WED	BREAKFAST:	DINNER:
	LUNCH:	SNACK:
THU	BREAKFAST:	DINNER:
	LUNCH:	SNACK:
FRI	BREAKFAST:	DINNER:
	LUNCH:	SNACK:
SAT	BREAKFAST:	DINNER:
	LUNCH:	SNACK:

WEEKLY MEAL PLAN JOURNAL

WEEK OF: _________

SUN	BREAKFAST:	DINNER:
	LUNCH:	SNACK:
MON	BREAKFAST:	DINNER:
	LUNCH:	SNACK:
TUE	BREAKFAST:	DINNER:
	LUNCH:	SNACK:
WED	BREAKFAST:	DINNER:
	LUNCH:	SNACK:
THU	BREAKFAST:	DINNER:
	LUNCH:	SNACK:
FRI	BREAKFAST:	DINNER:
	LUNCH:	SNACK:
SAT	BREAKFAST:	DINNER:
	LUNCH:	SNACK:

WEEKLY MEAL PLAN JOURNAL

WEEK OF: _________

SUN	BREAKFAST:	DINNER:
	LUNCH:	SNACK:
MON	BREAKFAST:	DINNER:
	LUNCH:	SNACK:
TUE	BREAKFAST:	DINNER:
	LUNCH:	SNACK:
WED	BREAKFAST:	DINNER:
	LUNCH:	SNACK:
THU	BREAKFAST:	DINNER:
	LUNCH:	SNACK:
FRI	BREAKFAST:	DINNER:
	LUNCH:	SNACK:
SAT	BREAKFAST:	DINNER:
	LUNCH:	SNACK:

BONUS 3: SHOPPING GUIDE

1.Know Your Triggers

Start by identifying foods high in salicylates that you need to avoid. Common culprits include certain fruits like berries, apples, and oranges, as well as vegetables like tomatoes and peppers. Also, be wary of spices such as curry, paprika, and thyme. Keeping a list of these high-salicylate foods on your phone or a small notepad can be a handy reference while shopping.

2. Read Labels Carefully

Packaged and processed foods often contain hidden salicylates, especially in flavourings, preservatives, and colorings. When you're at the store, take your time to read ingredient labels. Look out for terms like "natural flavours" or "spices," as these can sometimes include salicylates. Choosing products with minimal and clear ingredient lists will make it easier to avoid these hidden sources.

3. Focus on Low-Salicylate Foods

Build your shopping list around foods that are naturally low in salicylates. These include:

Grains: Rice, oats, and quinoa.
Dairy: Milk, cheese, and plain yoghurt.
Proteins: Most meats and poultry, eggs, and beans.
Vegetables: Cabbage, lettuce, and peas.
Fruits: Pears and bananas in moderation.

These foods will form the foundation of your meals and snacks, allowing you to enjoy a varied and balanced diet without the worry of triggering symptoms.

4. Explore Alternative Flavours

Spices and herbs high in salicylates are often staples in many recipes. Finding substitutes can keep your meals flavorful and exciting. Safe options include salt, fresh basil, and parsley. Experimenting with these can lead to delicious discoveries and help maintain the excitement in your cooking.

<u>**Practical Shopping Strategies**</u>

1.Shop the Perimeter

Fresh foods like produce, meat, and dairy are usually found around the perimeter of the store. These items are less likely to contain salicylates compared to the processed foods in the middle aisles. Focus on filling your cart with fresh, whole foods, which you can then prepare and season according to your dietary needs.

2.Buy in Bulk

For staples like rice, beans, and other grains, consider buying in bulk. Not only can this save you money, but it also reduces the need for frequent trips to the store, which can be time-consuming when you need to scrutinise every label. Bulk buying also means fewer chances of exposure to salicylates in packaging and preservatives.

<u>3.Visit Farmers' Markets</u>

Local farmers' markets often offer fresher and less processed options than big chain stores. This can be a great way to find high-quality, low-salicylate produce and meats. Plus, you can often speak directly with the growers and sellers to ask about their products and ensure they meet your dietary needs.

Additional Tips for a Successful Shopping Trip

Plan Ahead: Before you head to the store, take a few minutes to plan your meals and make a shopping list. This will help you stay focused and avoid impulse buys that might not be salicylate-safe.

Cook from Scratch: Preparing your meals from scratch gives you complete control over what goes into your food. This is the best way to avoid hidden salicylates and tailor your diet to your needs.

Stay Positive: Adjusting to a diet that avoids salicylates can be challenging, but it's also an opportunity to explore new foods and recipes.

Embrace the chance to get creative in the kitchen and discover flavours that work for you.

BONUS 4: FOOD LIST.

Low Salicylate Foods

These are the go-to foods for those with salicylate sensitivity. They contain minimal amounts of salicylates and are generally safe to consume in larger quantities.

Vegetables:
- Cabbage
- Celery
- Green beans
- Leeks
- Lettuce (iceberg)
- Potatoes (white)
- Swede (rutabaga)

Fruits:
- Pears (peeled)
- Golden Delicious apples (peeled)
- Bananas
- Papayas
- Watermelon

Protein:
- Beef
- Chicken (skinless)
- Eggs
- Fish (fresh, not canned or smoked)
- Lamb
- Pork

Grains and Carbs:
- White rice
- Plain pasta
- White bread
- Oats
- Cornflakes

Dairy:
- Milk
- Butter
- Cheese (mild varieties like cottage cheese)
- Yogurt (plain, without added fruits or flavours)

Beverages:

- Water
- Milk
- Pear juice
- Chamomile tea

Moderate Salicylate Foods

These foods have a moderate level of salicylates and can often be included in your diet in small amounts. They provide variety but should be consumed cautiously.

Vegetables:
- Broccoli
- Cauliflower
- Peas
- Pumpkin
- Sweet corn
- Zucchini

Fruits:
- Kiwi
- Mango
- Pineapple

- Avocado
- Raspberries

<u>Spices and Herbs:</u>
- Chives
- Parsley
- Rosemary
- Thyme

<u>Nuts and Seeds:</u>
- Macadamia nuts
- Sunflower seeds

<u>High Salicylate Foods</u>

These foods contain high levels of salicylates and are likely to trigger symptoms in sensitive individuals. It's best to avoid them or consume them only in very small quantities.

<u>Vegetables:</u>
- Spinach
- Eggplant
- Radishes

- Sweet potatoes
- Tomatoes

Fruits:

- Berries (strawberries, blueberries, blackberries)
- Grapes
- Oranges
- Apples (other than Golden Delicious)
- Cherries

Spices and Herbs:

- Cinnamon
- Curry powder
- Dill
- Oregano
- Turmeric

Nuts and Seeds:

- Almonds
- Peanuts
- Pistachios

Beverages:

- Coffee
- Tea (other than chamomile)
- Herbal teas with mixed ingredients
- Fruit juices (other than pear juice)

Hidden Sources of Salicylates

Salicylates can sneak into your diet through unexpected sources. Processed and packaged foods often contain additives derived from salicylates. Be cautious with the following:

- **Flavoured snacks**
- **Sauces and dressings**
- **Pre-packaged meals**
- **Soft drinks**
- **Certain candies and sweets**